# SEVERE CHRONIC COUGH REMEDY FOR ADULTS AND KIDS

By Smith J. Offor

# Table of Contents

# Introduction

## Organic Cough Remedies

### Honey

One or two teaspoons of honey may reduce mucus production. Germs are also killed by honey. But keep in mind that it can result in botulism, a rare form of food poisoning, in infants. Never give it to a kid who is under.

### Hot beverages

While hot drinks won't help with a stuffy head, they can help with a cough much more effectively than drinks that are room temperature. If you need relief, sip on hot tea or water.

## Ginger

According to research, ginger root's purified compounds can loosen up your airway's constricting muscles. Ginger can be consumed raw or combined with honey and stirred into hot tea.

## Water

The mucus in your throat becomes thinner when you drink lots of water, which also helps to soothe the scratch of a cough and keeps you hydrated. With a cough, you're less likely to need to clear things out.

## Steam

Because it soothes and moisturizes your airways, breathing in steam may help with coughing. For even more comfort, you can add a few drops of peppermint essential oil to the water.

## "Neti Pot."

Upper airway inflammation is one of the most typical causes of cough. Saline irrigation, which involves washing your nasal passages with saltwater, can reduce inflammation by flushing out irritants and removing mucus. Use a neti pot or a unique bulb.

## Elderberry

Elderberry extract is a dietary supplement that is available as a syrup or capsule. Even though it might not immediately make your cough better, studies show that it can hasten its resolution.

## Menthol

Your airways are naturally opened by the substance menthol, which is present in peppermint, making breathing easier.

Accordingly, it also has the ability to prevent coughs.

Menthol is an ingredient in cough drops, peppermint tea, and rubs that you apply to your chest.

## Use saltwater to gargle

Gargling with saltwater is typically used to treat sore throats, but it can also be effective for coughs. Much like a saline rinse does for the nose, the added moisture can help thin mucus and wash out things that irritate your throat. Tipping your head back while gargling, add 1/4 to 1/2 teaspoon of salt to 8 ounces of warm water. Then spit the solution out.

## Humidifier

While keeping the air moist can prevent a dry cough, use humidifiers with extra caution.

The leading cause of allergies is dust mites, which thrive in overly moist environments.

Furthermore, if humidifiers aren't kept clean, mold can develop inside of them. Both can exacerbate coughs rather than alleviate them.

## Herbs

Researchers have discovered that adding herbs like anise, ivy leaf, marshmallow root, and thyme to a syrup can reduce the number of days you'll experience a cough.

## Drops for coughing

Sucking on a cough drop or even just a hard candy may wet your throat sufficiently to temporarily stop coughing. Cough drops with menthol to open airways are your best option.

# 14 natural home remedies to treat a cough

1.

**Honey wax.**

Tea with honey and ginger is one of the best at-home treatments for a cough.

Drinking hot tea flavored with lemon and honey is the best home remedy for coughing.

Gargling with saltwater or consuming thyme are two additional natural cough remedies.

Invest in an air purifier or humidifier if your cough is dry, irritating, or allergy-related.

When something irritates your throat or airways, your body's natural reflex is to cough.

Coughing on occasion is normal and beneficial because it helps the body get rid of accumulated mucus and debris. They are still painful and exhausting despite this.

The following are the most typical causes of coughing:

• Anger caused by pollutants or sources like cigarette smoke.

• Bacterial infections, such as sinusitis and bronchitis.

1.

Allergies.

• asthma.

• Viral ailments like the cold or the flu.

Medical attention should be given to coughs brought on by allergies, infections, and asthma. To help you treat your cough at home, here are 13 suggestions if it persists after a viral infection or is brought on by irritation.

1.

## Select honey

High viscosity honey functions like a cough drop. When consumed, it coats the lining of the throat, reducing soreness or scratchiness. Dark honey, such as dark buckwheat honey, is more frequently studied for use in treating coughs than clover honey, which is more widely available.

Additionally, honey has anti-inflammatory, antioxidant, and antibacterial properties, which may help explain its calming effects. These qualities can strengthen your immune system and aid in the prevention of infections.

While honey can be eaten on its own, mixing it with hot tea can

enhance its throat-soothing
properties.

.

**Quick tip:** Honey should not be
given to children under the age of
one as it may contain bacteria that
cause infant botulism, a rare but
serious condition.

2.

## Use saltwater to gargle

Salt water gargling can aid in
removing mucus from your throat
and destroying bacteria. You can
clear your sinuses and get rid of
your cough more quickly by letting
go of the mucus in your throat. A
saltwater gargle can also aid in
easing the irritation and swelling
brought on by chronic coughing.

Cold water may also help your cough, despite the fact that most people prefer to gargle with warm salt water. Warm water, however, might hasten the salt's dissolution.

**Note**: For best results, season an eight-ounce glass of water with anywhere between 1/4 and 1/2 teaspoon of salt.

3.

## Ginger is an option

A common dietary supplement made from ginger is a tropical plant. The common cold, nausea, and the side effects of chemotherapy are just a few of the conditions it can help with.

The bioactive components in ginger have antioxidant, antimicrobial, and anti-inflammatory properties, just like those of honey. Additionally, ginger has a spicy flavor that increases salivation and helps treat dry mouth and sore throats.

People who have a cough may react differently to consuming spices, herbs, and spicy foods. It might help some people, but it might also aggravate their hacking and make it worse for others.

The most common way to consume ginger is as fresh or dried ginger root, but it can also be taken as a supplement in the form of a capsule or tincture. Try putting ginger and honey in your tea to help relieve your cough.

4.

## Inhale steam

Nasal congestion can be relieved by steam breathing. This will make blowing your nose simpler and, if you have post-nasal drip, release accumulated mucus in the throat. Steam may ease pain because it can moisturize a sore throat.

A boiling pot of water's steam can provide momentary relief. Take the water off the stove once it starts to steam, then stand in front of it. Put a towel over your head to help contain the steam, but watch out for getting too close or you could get burned. Taking a hot shower will also have a similar effect.

**A quick tip:** Stay away from the steam so that it is not coming in close contact with your skin in order to reduce the risk of burns.

5.

## Get a humidifier

A humidifier might also be a good choice if you live in a dry climate or during the winter to keep your sinuses clear. By releasing water vapor or steam into a space, humidifiers add moisture to the air.

How much space your humidifier will cover depends on its size.

If you do use a humidifier, make sure to regularly change the water and keep it clean to avoid unintentionally spreading mold or bacteria throughout your house.

# 6.

## Purchase a purifier for the air

Air purifiers assist in getting rid of allergens in your home that cause sneezing, coughing, and runny nose. In order to remove mold, bacteria, or dust, they circulate the air in your home through a number of filters, creating clean, fresh air.

Remember that air purifiers typically only work well in one room and to position it accordingly. In order for the filters to function properly, purifiers must also be regularly cleaned.

7.

## Utilize the marshmallow root

Inflammated mucous membranes in the mouth and throat are said to be calmed by the herbal supplement marshmallow root. Mucilage, a viscous substance, is found in the roots and leaves of marshmallow. Mucilage can coat the throat like honey when combined with water to create a texture that resembles gel.

Lozenges and marshmallow root extract were both effective in treating dry coughs, according to a 2018 study with over 800 participants that was published in Complementary Medicine Research. Within 10 minutes of taking the extract, the majority of participants noticed an improvement in their symptoms.

Dried marshmallow root leaves, teas, tinctures, and capsules are all available.

8.

## Eat thyme

Thyme is a herb that some people believe can relax smooth muscles, including coughing-related spasms. Thyme may have antifungal and antispasmodic properties that could aid in the treatment of infections and coughs.

90 percent of 750 cough patients in a German study from 2021 who were taking a thyme/ivy liquid

supplement reported a reduction in cough severity.

9.

## Hydrate yourself with water

Keeping hydrated is one of the simplest and safest ways to reduce your cough.

Mucus can leave the body through the mouth or nose by becoming thinner thanks to water consumption. Additionally, it can assist those who are ill in replacing fluids lost through sweating or a runny nose.

10.

## Consider probiotics

Live bacteria and other microorganisms are known as

probiotics, and they have been shown to have significant positive effects on gut health and digestion.

They can aid in restoring balance in your body, particularly when fighting an illness, when taken as a daily supplement or by increasing dietary intake of natural sources like yogurt and cheese.

11.

## Eat some pineapple

In addition to being delicious, pineapple is the best food to include in your diet if you want something healthy. By providing your body with vital vitamins and minerals thanks to the vitamin C, potassium, and magnesium it contains, pineapple helps to strengthen your immune system.

It is believed that pineapple helps to reduce inflammation in the respiratory system because it also contains bromelain, an enzyme known for its anti-inflammatory properties.

## 12.

## Consider slippery elm

Native Americans have long used slippery elm, an ingredient in the inner bark of the ulmusrubra tree, a common tree in North America, to treat sore throats, colds, and coughs.

The slippery and chewy texture of slippery elm gives it its name, and it also contains mucilage, a chemical that, when combined with water, increases the production of mucus, which soothes the throat and tissues around it.

## 13.

## Sip tea with peppermint

The healing properties of peppermint leaves are well known. The natural decongestant menthol found in peppermint, which is a component of peppermint, helps to clear mucus buildup and soothe sore throats.

Peppermint can also help you stay more hydrated when it is consumed as hot tea.

14.

## Use turmeric

Due to its well-known anti-inflammatory qualities, turmeric is used all over the world to treat a wide range of illnesses, including lung irritation, lung disease, and joint pain.

# 15 HOME CURE FOR A DRY COUGH

**How to cure a dry cough**

From over-the-counter and prescription medications to complementary treatments like raw honey and licorice root, there are many ways to get rid of a dry cough.

In contrast to a wet or productive cough, which produces mucus and phlegm, a dry cough does not produce any of these substances. The irritation of respiratory tract nerves that results from a dry cough can cause a scratchy or tickling sensation in the back of the throat.

The best way to treat a dry cough frequently depends on what caused it. Allergens, an infection, acid reflux, asthma, and nasal mucus are examples of what this could be.

## Dry cough home remedies in the kitchen

From one generation to the next, many treatments for treating the signs and symptoms of a dry cough have been passed down. There is frequently little more than anecdotal evidence to back their use, despite claims of effectiveness.

## Fresh honey

One of the most traditional home cures for any kind of cough is raw honey. It coats the throat and might have inbuilt anti-inflammatory qualities that can lessen throat irritation. Its potential antimicrobial effects may also lessen the severity of minor viral or bacterial infections.

Younger children generally tolerate honey well and enjoy it. However, due to the risk of botulism, it should never be given to infants younger than a year old. 3 If you need to be cautious about controlling your glucose levels, other options might be preferable because honey also affects blood sugar.

## Ginger

There is evidence that ginger, also known as Zingiberofficinale, may be effective in treating coughs in addition to nausea and upset stomach. By relaxing the smooth muscles in the airways, it is thought to prevent the reflex cough.

## Garlic

A mild antiviral, antibacterial, and anti-inflammatory compound is garlic (Allium sativum). Regular garlic consumption is also said to strengthen the immune system and lower blood pressure.

Although the results of the majority of studies looking into the effect have been conflicting, garlic is said to ease cough brought on by the common cold.

## Tumeric

Known as curcumin, turmeric (Curcuma longa) is thought to have tepid antiviral, antibacterial, and anti-inflammatory properties. 8 It has been used for thousands of years to treat respiratory conditions and mild arthritis in Ayurvedic medicine. However, the majority of these assertions are not backed up by research.

Researchers have hypothesized that taking turmeric orally may reduce asthma symptoms like coughing and other respiratory issues. Acute coughs have not been shown to benefit from it.

In light of the aforementioned, turmeric tea is widely available in grocery stores and is generally well-tolerated. The problem with turmeric capsules is that if you take too much of the supplement, you might get nauseated, have diarrhea, and upset your stomach.

## Water containing salt

Healthcare professionals frequently advise gargling with saltwater to relieve a sore throat and cough brought on by the common cold. In order to lessen inflammation and swelling, saltwater draws moisture away from the sore area.

## Hydration

Your cough could get worse if you have a dry throat. Drinking water, honey-and-lemon tea, and herbal teas are all good options.

The following herbal teas can be useful for a dry cough.

- Ginger
-  The licorice root.
- marjoram.
- "Marshmallow root.".
-  Masala Chai.
- Peppermint.
- Thyme.
- Turmeric.

**Over-the-Counter Treatments for Dry Cough**
When you are recovering from a cold, OTC treatments can frequently help you with your cough.

## Drops for coughing

When you have a cough and sore throat, cough drops are frequently sufficient to provide relief. Choose lozenges with menthol, which has a cooling effect and serves as a light anesthetic.

To further ease your discomfort, mix a mentholated product, such as Vicks Vapo-Rub, into your steam inhalation.

## Drugs for coughing

Dry cough is frequently treated with dextromethorphan, an over-the-counter drug.

You can use a generic version, and popular brands include:

- Cough from Delsym.

- Robitussin Cough.

Remember that many OTC cough medications also act as decongestants; if your cough is dry, you may not require this effect.

Call the office of your healthcare provider to discuss your symptoms and get their advice. Your pharmacist might be able to provide you with guidance regarding over-the-counter medications.

## Steam therapies

By inhaling steam, you might be able to cure your dry cough. Warm steam can soothe sore throats, moisten dry and irritated nasal passages, and lessen the severity of a cough brought on by a minor infection or allergy.

You can inhale more moisture by covering your head with a towel as you take a breath of the steam. A severe burn could result if you put your face close to a pot of boiling water.

If you don't want to do it yourself, you can purchase a steam inhaler from a pharmacy or online.

Are You Sleepless at Night Due to Dry Cough?

Try the following to find the relaxation and relief you require:

Consuming some liquids before bed, such as warm tea.

Using additional pillows to elevate your head can help prevent acid reflux and throat irritation from nasal drip.

If the air feels dry while you're trying to sleep, try running a cool-mist humidifier.

## Herbal Treatments for Dry Coughs

It may be reasonable to treat your dry cough at home if it is mild and uncomplicated, that is, if there is no fever, chest pain, or any other alarming symptoms.

### Liqueur Root

There has long been talk about the throat-soothing benefits of drinking licorice root (Glycyrrhiza glabra) tea. Licorice root has been used since 2100 B.C., when it was known as gancao in traditional Chinese medicine and is thought to ease cough, clear phlegm, and lessen pain.

There are lots of grocery and health food stores where you can buy licorice root tea. Dried licorice root can be purchased online and used to make tea by steeping 2 tablespoons of the shaved root in 8 ounces of boiling water for five to 10 minutes. Even though prolonged use of licorice root tea is generally thought to be safe, it can also result in menstrual irregularities, fatigue, headaches, water retention, and erectile dysfunction in addition to sharp increases in blood pressure.

# Marjoram

Traditional medicine has long relied on marjoram (Origanummajorana), a variety of oregano, to treat a variety of ailments. It is rumored to contain anti-inflammatory, plant-based compounds (phytochemicals) that could lessen cough brought on by pertussis (whooping cough), bronchitis, colds, and asthma.

Three to four teaspoons of dried marjoram should be steeped in eight ounces of hot water to make marjoram tea, which should be consumed three times per day.

Marjoram is generally regarded as being safe, but in people who are taking anticoagulant (blood-thinning) medications, it may slow blood clotting and increase the risk of bruising and nosebleeds.

## "Marshmallow Root.".

According to its name, marshmallow root is the root of the hollyhock plant known as the marshmallow plant (Althea officinalis).

Since ancient times, marshmallow root has been used to soothe sore throats, frequently in the form of a sweet, meringue-like treat. Its slightly gooey texture can soothe scratchy throats, and the flavonoids in the root are thought to reduce inflammation.

A 2018 study published in Complementary Medicine Research found that marshmallow root extract was used to make syrups and lozenges that provided mild dry cough relief, typically within 10 minutes.

Online and in a few specialty health food stores, marshmallow root tea can be purchased. Despite the fact that not much research has been done to evaluate its long-term safety, it is generally regarded as safe.

Blood clotting and blood sugar levels may be impacted by the plant.


## Thyme

Since the Black Plague infected Europe, thyme (Thymus vulgaris) has been used medicinally. It includes a substance called thymol, which is thought to have antispasmodic properties that can help soothe the smooth muscles in the throat.

Thyme is probably safe to use occasionally when prepared as tea. 3–4 teaspoons of the dried herb can be infused in 8 ounces of boiling water to create thyme tea. Add honey to the sweetness for additional cough-relieving benefits.

Because it can cause a potentially dangerous drop in blood pressure, thyme essential oil, which is typically used in aromatherapy, should not be consumed internally.

## Basil the Holy

Holy basil, also known as tulsi, is a green-leafed plant that is indigenous to India. Its scientific name is Ocimum tenuiflorum. It has been utilized for a number of things for thousands of years, including the treatment of a dry cough.

Holy basil is generally safe to use, but there is little scientific research on its effectiveness.

You can add holy basil extract to make it into tea or steam it.

## Aromatherapy

Inhaling plant extracts or essential oils for therapeutic purposes is known as aromatherapy. You have the choice of applying them topically, diffusing them into the air with an essential oil diffuser, or using an aroma stick.

The following are some examples
of essential oils that may soothe a
dry cough.


- Eucalyptus
- Holy Basil
- Peppermint
- Thyme

It's critical to use essential oils
safely because they can have
strong effects and differing effects
on different people. You can get
assistance from a healthcare
professional in selecting the
options that might work best for
you.

# The use of essential oils for asthma

## What Leads to Dry Coughing?

Everything from indoor air quality to medical conditions can irritate the throat and result in a chronic dry cough.

## Interior Air Quality

The dryness of colder air can cause a dry cough because it is typically drier. Some airborne irritants, such as smoke, pollen, dander, and dust, can cause a dry cough in some people.

You can take a number of steps at home to prevent your environment from causing or aggravating your cough:

**Use a cool-mist humidifier:** If
your coughing tends to worsen in
dry weather, a humidifier can help
by introducing moisture to the air
to alleviate your dry cough. When
you can, especially at night, use
one.

Use an air purifier to remove dust,
dander, and pollen from the air,
which can help people with
allergies and irritants. If you suffer
from asthma, this may be useful.

**Don't smoke**: Smoke from
cigarettes, vaporizers, and
marijuana causes more throat
irritation.

## Medicine-Related Causes

Allergies, irritants in the
environment, infections, and even
some medications (like ACE

inhibitors) can all result in a dry cough.

A chronic cough could be a first indication of a health problem like sleep apnea or gastroesophageal reflux disease (GERD).


The following medical conditions can also result in a dry cough:.

Seasonal hay fever and indoor allergies can both result in a dry cough.

When pollen and mold counts start to rise, taking an oral antihistamine daily can help prevent allergies.

**Asthma:** Asthma, particularly cough-variant asthma, can cause a dry cough. It is possible to lessen the frequency of attacks by taking your asthma medications as prescribed, including long-acting bronchodilators and inhaled corticosteroids.

A dry cough may be brought on by acid reflux. An acid blocker can help, as can staying away from high-fat, acidic, chocolate, caffeine-containing, and spicy foods, all of which can make your symptoms worse.

Side effects of taking certain medications include a dry cough. Coughing may be triggered by ACE inhibitors, Fluticasone nasal sprays, Coreg (carvedilol), Zocor (simvastatin), Actonel (risedronate), and Zocor (simvastatin). When dealing with this frequent side effect, it may be sufficient to reduce the dosage or switch medications. Just make sure to first check with your doctor.

# PERSISENT COUGH

**Diagnosis**
However, rather than recommending costly tests, many doctors choose to begin treating one of the common causes of chronic cough. You might, however, be tested for less typical causes if the medication doesn't work.

- Imaging examinations
- X-rays

The most frequent causes of a cough, postnasal drip, acid reflux, and asthma, are not revealed by a routine chest X-ray, but it can be used to test for lung cancer, pneumonia, and other lung diseases. Evidence of a sinus infection may be seen on an X-ray of your sinuses.

CT scans performed using a computer. Additionally, CT scans may be used to examine your sinus cavities for pockets of infection or your lungs for conditions that could result in a chronic cough.

- Tests of lung function.
- Spirometer.
- Boost image size

Asthma and COPD are diagnosed using these straightforward, non-invasive tests, such as spirometry. Both your ability to hold and exhale quickly are measured.

When you take the medication methacholine (Provocholine), your doctor may order an asthma challenge test to see how well you can breathe both before and after.

## Tests in the lab

Your doctor might want to check a sample of the mucus you cough up for bacteria if it is colored.

## Scope assessments

If your doctor is unable to identify the cause of your cough, specialized scope tests to look for potential causes may be considered. These examinations could consist of:

## Bronchoscopy

Your doctor can examine your lungs and airways using a bronchoscope, a thin, flexible tube outfitted with a light and camera. To check for anomalies, a biopsy can also be performed on the mucosa that lines the interior of your airway.

## Rhinoscopy

Your doctor can see your nasal passages, sinuses, and upper airway using a fiberoptic scope (rhinoscope).

To identify the cause of a persistent cough in children, a chest X-ray and spirometry are typically ordered.

## Treatment

For a chronic cough to be effectively treated, the cause must be identified. Frequently, your chronic cough may be brought on by a number of underlying conditions.

If you smoke, your doctor will talk to you about whether you're ready to stop and offer support in doing so.

If you are currently taking an ACE inhibitor, your doctor may switch you to a different drug that doesn't have cough as a side effect.

The following medicines may be used to treat chronic cough:

Corticosteroids, decongestants, and antihistamines. For postnasal drip and allergies, these medications are standard care.

Drugs for asthma inhaled. Corticosteroids and bronchodilators, which decrease inflammation and widen your airways, are the best treatments for cough associated with asthma.

## Antibiotics

In the event that a bacterial, fungal, or mycobacterial infection is the root of your persistent cough, your doctor may recommend antibiotics to treat the infection.

a acid blocker. Acid-blocking medications may be prescribed to you if lifestyle modifications are ineffective in treating your acid reflux. Some people require surgery to solve their issues.

## Antitussive drugs

Your doctor may also prescribe a cough suppressant in an effort to hasten the symptom relief process while they identify the cause of your cough and start treatment.

The goal of over-the-counter cough and cold medications is to alleviate symptoms, not the underlying illness. According to research, it hasn't been demonstrated that these medications are any more effective than a placebo. More importantly, these drugs may have harmful side effects, such as fatal overdoses in children under the age of two.

Children younger than 6 years old should not be treated for coughs and colds with over-the-counter medications, with the exception of painkillers and fever reducers. Additionally, think twice before giving these medications to kids under the age of 12.

**Lifestyle and DIY remedies**
Take the advice your doctor gives you regarding how to treat the cause of your cough. You can also attempt these suggestions in the interim to reduce your cough:

Drink plenty of liquids to help your throat's mucus thin out. Your throat can feel better after drinking warm liquids like broth, tea, or juice.

Cough drops or hard candies should be sucked. They might relieve a dry cough and calm an abrasive throat.

Take honey into consideration. A teaspoon of honey could ease a cough. Children under the age of one should not be given honey because it may contain bacteria that are harmful to young children.

Use a cool-mist humidifier or take a steamy shower to moisturize the air.

## Prevent using tobacco

Your lungs become irritated when you smoke or breathe secondhand smoke, which can make any existing coughing fits worse. If you smoke, discuss products and programs with your doctor that can help you stop.

## Cough: What Is It?

The reflexive action of coughing aids in clearing mucus, foreign objects, and irritants from the throat and airways. Allergies, environmental factors, viral or bacterial infections, as well as some medications, can all contribute to coughing. Wheezing, breathing issues, tightness in the chest, sore throat, fever, and chills are all signs of a cough.

The brain receives a signal from the body when it coughs, which causes a reflex action. The diaphragm muscles contract first, causing a sharp exhalation. Air is expelled through the mouth and nose at the same time that the vocal cords close to produce a "coughing" sound. Coughing is a reliable method of clearing the airways of unwelcome substances because the air exhaled through the mouth and nose also aids in clearing any mucus or irritants in the throat and lungs.

## Various Coughing Patterns

An ineffective cough that produces no phlegm or mucus is referred to as a "dry cough.". It frequently happens when environmental factors like smoke, dust, or cold air irritate the throat and airways.

Wet Cough: Also referred to as a productive cough, this type of cough results in the production of mucus or phlegm that is then coughed up. This kind of cough can be brought on by bacterial or viral infections, allergies, bronchitis, asthma, and other conditions.

A spasmodic cough is a severe, intermittent coughing fit that can last for a few minutes. It is frequently brought on by irritation of the respiratory mucous membrane, which causes involuntary muscle contractions, which in turn cause the spasmodic coughing.

## Natural Remedies for Cough Relief

Coughs, as we now know, are one of the most widespread illnesses and can be painful and irritating.

The good news is that there are many effective natural remedies that can help to relieve a cough and permanently end it.

Drinking plenty of fluids is one of the easiest things you can do. This will aid in thinning mucus and make it simpler for your body to eliminate it. Honey is a fantastic cough suppressant and is thought to have antibacterial properties.

Gargling with salt water is another effective treatment because it helps to break down mucus, which makes it easier to expel and lessens throat inflammation.

Gargle with a solution made by combining honey and lemon juice for a stronger cure. For relieving a ticklish cough, this mixture can be especially helpful.

Consider using a steam inhalation if your cough is especially persistent. This entails pouring freshly boiled water into a bowl and spending around ten minutes inhaling the steam through your nose. Repeating this several times per day can assist in re-loosening mucus and facilitating its expulsion. The effectiveness of the steam can also be increased by adding a few drops of eucalyptus essential oil or a few spoonfuls of salt.

There are a lot of herbal teas available as well that can soothe a cough. For instance, ginger tea is regarded as a potent natural remedy. Thyme, licorice root, and marshmallow root are some additional herbs that are frequently used. Another option is elderberry syrup.

## Top 8 Homeopathic Cough Treatments.

Aconite is a fundamental component of any homeopathic first aid kit.

At the first sign of a cough, especially if it begins after being exposed to chilly, dry winds, aconite is administered. For this reason, we also give aconite to people whose coughs started after a cough or fright (terror and fear are a big part of the aconite picture). However, coughs might not start because of an environmental factor; they can also be triggered by emotional events. If a person also has a high fever, chills, shivering, anxiety, or a feeling of impending doom, aconite may be the right treatment.

The aconite cough is a hoarse, dry, and croupy cough that gets worse at night and makes you want to go outside and relax. Additionally, the cough gets better in the fresh air and gets worse after drinking cold water.

# Keynotes for Aconia.

- Conditions caused by dry, chilly winds, becoming extremely cold, and shock.
- High fever or a cold with chills may accompany coughing.
- shivering.
- A croupy, dry cough that is hoarse.
- Starts around midnight or worsens afterward.
- Anxiety, a sense of great unease, and tossing and turning.
- A sense of impending death.
- A tickly throat with a dry, suffocating cough.
- Barking cough and croup.

- Cold water consumption is worse at night and after midnight.
- More beneficial for resting outside.

## Everything is dry and painful, according to Bryonia.

The hard, dry, hacking cough that distinguishes bryonia is characterized by a slow, gradual onset and is brought on by irritation in the upper trachea (windpipe). Bryonia cough patients experience stabbing pains in the sides of their chest as they cough. They may have to hold their chest while coughing because the cough is so painful, and if they are lying down, they will naturally sit up.

Dryness (very little phlegm) and the desire to remain still are the hallmarks of a bryonian cough. The cough is aggravated by talking, laughing, or moving; it is also worse at night and in warm settings. The person frequently feels extremely thirsty and drinks large amounts of liquid in gulps. They may feel better with hard pressure on the chest or in cool, open air. A bryonia cough causes a dry, painful cough, which makes the person likely to be very irritable and want privacy.

Bryonia is a fantastic treatment for coughs that are dry, painful, thirsty, and irritable, to sum up.

**Keynotes by Bryonia:**
- slowly building up.

- An irritable upper trachea causes a hard, dry, hacking cough.
- Dry, hard, and extremely painful holding the chest still and relieving the pain.
- Sharp, stabbing chest pains and soreness are brought on by coughing.
- dryness and scant mucus production.
- Unwillingly getting out of bed or a chair in response to a cough.
- Worse for movement, speaking, laughing, entering a warm room, inspiration, and night.
- Better for rest, hard pressure, lying on the painful side, cold things, and cool open air.
- irritable and needs solitude.

- big gulps of liquid when extremely thirsty.

**Spongia.**
Similar to bryonia, the spongia cough is abrasive, dry, and barking. Like a foghorn, the cough has a deep, hollow sound. It is worse for inspiration, which is particularly annoying when coughing because, after a coughing fit, you typically need to take a deep breath of air to catch your breath and you can end up in a vicious circle. Before midnight, when the cough is at its worst, the person may choke on it while sleeping and experience anxiety about suffocating.

The cough may feel as though the person's chest is about to explode and may result in burning sensations in the throat, larynx, and chest. Additionally, the airways are dry, and the person might feel as though they are breathing through a sponge.

The good news is that, in contrast to acontie, the spongia cough may get better after eating or drinking, especially warm beverages. Additionally, they might experience relief by bending forward or by sucking on something sweet. Right-side lying and bending the head may help with the cough.

Although similar, spongia's therapeutic modalities are distinct from those of aconite, a drug used

to treat fear. Spongia is
considerably less anxious.

## Keynotes from Spongia:

- Foghorn coughs are rough, dry, barking, croupy, deep, and hollow.
- Breathing problems are worse before midnight and during inspiration.
- After coughing, there is burning in the throat, larynx, and chest; the chest feels as though it might rupture.
- Following eating and drinking, especially warm beverages, coughing often occurs.

- Deep, raw, and painful spot in the chest; dryness in all airways.
- feels like "breathing through a sponge.".
- Coughs have a "dry as a bone" sound, akin to a saw cutting through a pine board or "Seals bark.".
- anxiety and fear of suffocation while falling asleep and choking.
- Talking is more difficult when it's dry, windy, before midnight, physically demanding, drinking cold beverages, or lying on one's right side.
- Better for warming up food or beverages for consumption, sucking on candies, swallowing, and bending the head forward.

- deeper and less frightful than aconite!

**Drosera.**

A dry, irritable, and spasmodic cough that is specific to the drosera species is present. The cough can be so severe that the sufferer worries they won't be able to breathe. Considering how much they are coughing, they might even retch and vomit. It can begin as soon as the person's head touches the pillow at night and is a deep, hoarse cough.

In a manner similar to bryonia, but without the pain that comes along with it, the person may hold their chest while coughing, and they may experience throat tightness or a tickling sensation that makes them cough. The cough usually gets worse in the evening, right before bedtime, and in stuffy places. They may also produce yellow phlegm.

When in the open air, sitting up in bed, moving around, or relaxing quietly, someone with a drosera cough will feel better.

**The Keynotes of Drosera.**
• A rapid succession of dry, irritable, spasmodic coughs that make it difficult to breathe out completely.

• Rapid, persistent coughing may cause nausea and vomiting.

• Deep, hoarse, barking, or choking sounds when coughing.

• The heat of the bed causes a cough to begin as soon as the head touches the pillow.

• When a cough feels tight (like Bryonia's did), the person holds their chest.

• Tickling in the back of the throat; possible presence of yellow phlegm from the cough.

• Worse for lying down, conversing, in the evening after midnight, stuffy room.

• Sitting up in bed, motion, and quietness are better for pressure and open air.

## Ant Tart, which means "Mucus, Mucus, and More Mucus!".

Children who frequently contract chest colds with a wet, mucus-filled cough will benefit greatly from this treatment.

Due to the accumulation of mucus in the chest, an ant tart cough causes a loud rattling noise that makes the person sound almost as though they are drowning. Even though there is a lot of mucus, the person might have trouble coughing it up. Due to the amount of mucus produced by the cough, which is similar to drosera but is a dry cough, breathing becomes difficult, and the person may even vomit. After a coughing fit, the person may feel worn out and sleepy and the mucus has a thick, white, ropey appearance.

On the emotional side of things, when someone has a cough that could use a few doses of ant tart, they might not like to be looked at or spoken to. In warm, stuffy spaces, they'll feel worse, and anger or other strong emotions could make things worse. If at all possible, sit upright in a cool room with a window open and leave them alone. In the case of a child, they might also be in need of parental support and have a thirst for cold water.

**Keynotes by Ant Tart:**
• Kids who frequently catch chest-flush-producing colds.

• A choking cough that produces copious amounts of rattling mucus, but very little expectoration.

• Seem to be drowning and unable to raise phlegm.

• Thick, loose, rattling cough; chest feels mucus-filled.

• Because of the phlegm on the chest, breathing is challenging.

• Thick, ropy, white mucus that is vomited after coughing.

• Must sit up because they feel like they're going to suffocate.

• After coughing fit, may seem worn out and sleepy.

• Worse for touching, eating, lying down, eating in hot, stuffy rooms, being looked at, and for cold, wet weather.

• Lying on the right side, being cold, outside, sitting up, vomiting, expectoration, and being left alone are all better.

## HeparSulph.

Heparsulph, a homeopathic remedy like aconite, is used to treat symptoms brought on by exposure to cold, more specifically dry cold. Particularly for dry coughs or coughs with thick yellow mucus, this remedy is advised.

The person in need of this remedy may be easily agitated and extremely sensitive to cold air, especially in the morning. In addition to preferring warm beverages, they will feel better in a warm room covered in blankets. It's important to keep in mind that because these people are so sensitive to drafts, getting them out of bed and giving them a cool drink won't go over well. When someone coughs, they might feel as though there is a splinter in their throat, and they might need to bend their head backwards in order to cough.

Sincerity dictates that when someone has a heparsulph cough, it's best to leave them alone, wrap them in blankets, and avoid bothering them unless it's to bring them a warm beverage.

# Keynotes for HeparSulph:

• Cough brought on by exposure to the cold, particularly dry, chilly air, and west or northwest winds.

• Once chilled, can be exacerbated by exposure to a cold draft.

• A cough that is loose, rattling, or noisy and produces thick, yellow mucus.

• A croupy, choking cough necessitates standing up and bending the head back.

• Coughing is brought on by a sensation of a fish bone or splinter in the throat.

• Feels extremely cold, is extremely susceptible to a draft, or feels colder than usual; coughing may result from taking a hand out of bedclothes.

• Extremely irritable, overly sensitive, and disinterested in attention.

• Worse for cold air, early mornings, any part of the body getting cold or exposed, walking, eating, or drinking anything cold.

Better wrapped up and heated in a warm environment.


**Phosphorus.**
A really violent and dry cough that would benefit from some phosphorus supplements. The burning sensation in the throat, along with dryness and tickling, is the defining feature of a phosphorus cough. The environment, including the

weather and temperature, can affect how well this remedy works. The change in climate is what makes this cough worse; the symptoms will be the same in windy, dry, and cold weather as they will in wet, hot weather.

Phosphorus is also prone to a hot sensation in the chest, a dry cough, and headache pain. Sleeping is made challenging by the cough, which is frequently hollow and occurs mostly in the morning and at night. If present, phlegm may contain a trace amount of blood.

Phosphorus-deficient individuals experience anxiety and fear and yearn for companionship and understanding. Particularly if they are young, they need to be reassured and comforted. They enjoy cold beverages and ice cream.

The right side of the bed, talking, laughing, and dusk all make this remedy worse.

**Keynotes on phosphorus.**

• A harsh, dry cough that causes throat tickling and burning dryness.

• The weather changing, being windy and cold, and getting wet in the heat.

• Every cold ends with a cough or spreads to the chest.

• A burning sensation behind the sternum and a hot sensation in the chest.

• A dry cough coupled with a throbbing headache.

• A hollow cough, which is most common in the morning in bed but can also occur at night, keeps people from falling asleep.

• Morning phlegm can be transparent or blood-stained.

• Needs support and sympathy and is fearful and anxious.

• Worse for talking, laughing, lying on the left side, evening, and twilight.

• Better for massages, touch, sitting up when coughing, lying on the right side, and cold beverages.

## Pulsatilla.

Getting wet outside, especially if their feet become completely submerged, can cause pulsatilla symptoms to appear. This remedy can be emotionally triggered by grief or abandonment.

A pulsatilla cough frequently worsens at dusk and feels better after touching or massaging it, especially when upright. They must stand up to cough, but they feel better lying on their right side.

Their primary characteristic is a cough that can be loose in the morning and dry in the evening, but they also enjoy cold beverages.

Usually accompanied by a runny
nose with thick yellow or green
discharge, the cough is rattling
and produces thick yellow mucus.

Someone who needs pulsatilla for
a cough will crave love and
sympathy and feel very
withdrawn, tearful, and clingy.
Both the evening dry cough and
the morning loose cough make
them worse. They dislike stuffy
rooms and favor open, cool air.
Even though they might feel better
with cold beverages, they
frequently lack thirst and may
need encouragement to drink.

**Keynotes of the Pulsatilla.**

• Illnesses brought on by grief, being abandoned, getting cold, or wet feet.

• Symptoms that fluctuate, e.g. loose in the morning and dry at night.

• A rattling cough accompanied by profuse, thick yellow mucus and a runny nose.

• A short, dry, hacking cough brought on by epigastric tickling.

• A dry cough, headache, and nausea.

• Demands sympathy and attention, is withdrawn, clingy and weepy, and is wingy and whiny.

• Worse in the morning (loose), evening (dry), and when left alone, as well as in warm environments and stuffy spaces.

• Better for rubbing and massaging, sitting up straight with your head held high, and enjoying cool, fresh, open air.

These medications should be a part of any good remedy kit and can be purchased at health food stores or homeopathic pharmacies.

## When And How To Use Your Treatment.

When selecting a treatment, think about the symptoms and distinguish between treatment modalities, as well as what makes the symptoms better or worse and any supplementary symptoms.

Of course, it's best to see a doctor if your cough is particularly severe or if your symptoms continue. These treatments can be helpful, but it's crucial to apply them correctly.

# Five natural home remedies for a long-lasting dry cough!

People of all ages can be seen with a dry cough, making it a common ailment. A chronic cough without mucus or phlegm is what distinguishes it from other coughs. For the treatment of dry cough, there are many over-the-counter options available, but some people prefer to use natural home remedies. We will examine at-home treatments for dry cough in this article.

How can a dry cough be treated?

## 1. Mulethi, also known as licorice root.

Mulethi is known to calm irritated airways because of its anti-inflammatory and expectorant properties. According to a study that appeared in the Journal of Pharmaceutical Biology, patients with chronic obstructive pulmonary disease (COPD) who take licorice root extract report fewer coughs and improved respiratory symptoms. The research suggests that mulethi may be a helpful treatment for COPD-related dry cough. Simply place a small piece of mulethi in your mouth and continue to chew it.

For a dry cough, use mulethi.

It will relieve your throat pain whether you chew on it raw or drink mulethi tea. Image courtesy of Shutterstock.

## 2. Honey.

You cannot discuss cough treatment without mentioning honey. Honey is a natural remedy for dry cough because it eases throat discomfort and suppresses coughing. According to a study in the journal Pediatrics, dextromethorphan, a common component of over-the-counter cough medicines, is less effective at treating children's coughs than honey.

### 3. Ginger.

Ginger has anti-inflammatory qualities and is well known for relieving airway irritation. In patients with acute bronchitis, ginger is effective at reducing cough and throat pain. When it comes to treating a dry cough, ginger may be helpful. To sooth your throat when you have a dry cough, make a cup of honey-ginger spiced tea.

### 4. Intake of steam.

By moistening the airways, steam inhalation is a straightforward home remedy that can help relieve dry cough. Inhaling steam helped patients with cough symptoms and required fewer medications, according to a study that was published in the International Journal of Chronic Obstructive Pulmonary Disease. It is among the best methods for clearing your airways of all the irritants that are the cause of your dry cough.

**5. Gargle with salt water.** Dry cough can be treated by gargling with lukewarm saltwater 2 to 3 times per day. According to a study in the American Journal of Preventive Medicine, healthy adults who gargle with saltwater have fewer respiratory infections overall. The study makes the case for salt water gargling as a potential treatment for dry cough brought on by respiratory infections.

# Chronic cough syndrome signs and diagnosis.

Most people have experienced a cough at some point in their lives.

Coughing has many causes and is a very common symptom. Common causes of coughing include viral upper respiratory infections, lung disease, heart failure, reflux, choking on food or other foreign objects in your throat, adverse effects of some medications, exposure to airway irritants like tobacco smoke, pollutants, or perfumes, and habit. More serious issues like pneumonia, cancer, and uncommon lung conditions are less frequent causes. However, most coughing is self-limiting and doesn't last more than a week or two.

Coughs that last longer than six weeks are typically considered to be part of chronic cough syndrome. People with chronic coughing frequently have multiple causes at play.

Depending on the cause(s) of the cough, chronic cough syndrome may be accompanied by other symptoms. Heartburn or indigestion, wheezing (whistling sounds) or shortness of breath (including a challenge taking a deep breath in or out) are a few of these.

"Chest congestion," as described by some patients.

Additionally, sneezing, nasal congestion, nasal drainage, and a "drip," or drainage down the back of your throat, can all be brought on by coughing.

It's crucial to start by speaking with your allergist or immunologist to identify the root cause or causes of your persistent cough. In order to ascertain whether your cough is being accompanied by any other symptoms, your allergist will take a thorough medical history. It's crucial that you inform your allergist or immunologist about and bring any medications you're taking, including prescription, over-the-counter, vitamins, supplements, herbal remedies, and homeopathic remedies. The physical examination can be beneficial as well. The tests that will be required to identify the cause(s) of the cough will be determined by the results of these preliminary steps, if any.

## The management of investigations.

The cause of chronic cough syndrome is diagnosed using a variety of techniques. Given that allergic rhinitis and the resulting post-nasal drip are a significant contributor to chronic cough, allergy testing can help identify any inhalant allergens to which you are allergic (such as mold, dust mites, mold, grass, or weed pollens). An allergist should be consulted when ordering, carrying out, and interpreting allergy tests. Limiting triggers for allergies and irritants in the home and workplace might be important. Masks can shield the airways from irritating chemicals and dangerous substances.

A chronic cough can be caused by a variety of lung conditions. Your allergist or immunologist can diagnose asthma, a common condition that can cause wheezing, coughing, and shortness of breath. Your allergist or immunologist may use lung or breathing tests to identify the source of your cough. A chest x-ray and a CT ("CAT") scan of your sinuses are examples of radiological tests. A laryngoscopy, a procedure that can be done in the doctor's office using a tube, or "scope," to look inside your nasal cavities and throat, may be one of the additional tests you undergo. .

Reflux is another name for gastroesophageal reflux disease (GERD), which can cause heartburn or indigestion symptoms. The chronic cough syndrome can be exacerbated by and caused by this. It's important to keep in mind that you might only have a cough and not even experience or feel heartburn. While there are specific procedures available to diagnose GERD, your allergist or immunologist may frequently put you on a GERD medication for a specific amount of time while they watch to see if your cough symptoms get better. .

In collaboration with your hypertension doctor, your allergist or immunologist may change your high blood pressure medication to see if your cough gets better.

Certain high blood pressure (hypertension) medications, such as ACE inhibitors (lisinopril, for instance), can cause chronic cough syndrome.

Finally, many patients can profit from therapies to lessen throat sensitivity, known as cough hypersensitivity syndrome, if diagnostic testing and management of these common conditions are ineffective (e. g. habit cough), which can cause coughing. In these circumstances, your allergist might suggest speech therapy or bring up the possibility of using suppressing therapy in conjunction with particular medications to lessen coughing fits.

## Treatment

Depending on the cause or suspected cause(s) of chronic cough syndrome, there are numerous treatment options available. These include inhalers, nasal sprays, and oral medications (liquids and tablets). It should be noted that many popular over-the-counter drugs have limitations in that they frequently do not treat the precise cause(s) of the cough. A chronic cough should not be treated with drugs like codeine due to the risk of addiction. Codeine is specifically not advised for acute or persistent cough in children due to safety concerns. .

Some people have multiple medical issues, which could be a factor in their chronic cough. As a result, managing your symptoms frequently involves a

multidisciplinary approach
involving the collaboration of
gastroenterologists, allergists,
pulmonologists, speech therapists,
and otorhinolaryngologists.

Children, toddlers, and babies can
cough from 8 different types.

**Symptoms:** According to Dr.
Berger, your child may experience
a cough and a low-grade fever as a
result of the virus. Some children
are unable to cough the mucus out
as the congestion worsens, so they
choose to swallow it. All that
mucus can also upset a child's
stomach or cause them to gag,
which may result in them puking.
He continues by saying that,
following a cold, the cough may

last much longer than the runny
nose.

**Treatment:** The majority of the
time, a cold needs to pass on its
own. Cough and cold remedies are
not advised for children under the
age of six, according to the
American Academy of Pediatrics.
To treat a child's persistent cough
brought on by a cold, try the
following home remedies.

Give your child plenty of fluids,
including popsicles, warm
decaffeinated tea, and water.
Avoid citrus juice and carbonated
beverages as they can irritate your
throat.

At night, turn on a cool-mist
humidifier or vaporizer; the

moisture will aid in clearing his airways.

To relieve nasal congestion, use a suction syringe or saline nasal spray.

Offer 1/2 to 1 teaspoon of honey in tea or on toast to children older than 1 year old as needed to help with coughing.

Carrie Quinn, M.D says, "Parents frequently worry when a cough is persistent, especially when it sounds harsh. , a pediatrician at New York City's Mount Sinai Kravis Children's Hospital. "However, there are inquiries you ought to make to ascertain the severity of the cough. A healthcare provider should be consulted if the cough persists after two to three weeks or if your child exhibits

breathing issues, vomiting, or a
spike in fever.

**Sinusitis.**
If your child's cough won't go away
and lasts for more than ten days,
they might have sinusitis. This is
an inflammation of the mucus
lining of the sinuses and nose. The
result is a persistent cough and a
thick, yellowish-green nasal
discharge. It also causes air
pockets to form along the brow,
cheekbones, and nose. As
congestion worsens, sinuses turn
into a breeding ground for
bacteria.

# 9 Homeopathic Treatments for Toddler Cough.

Symptoms: In addition to a persistent cough, sinusitis can result in postnasal drip, bad breath, fatigue, eye puffiness, and dark circles. Children who are older may also experience headaches. Children can develop a seemingly never-ending, persistent cough from even a mild sinus infection.

**Treatment:** To combat the infection and relieve symptoms, a primary care physician may recommend an antibiotic and nasal sprays. After a few days, if your child doesn't seem to be getting better, they might require another round of antibiotics or another type of medication. To relieve headaches or facial pain, try acetaminophen, ibuprofen, or warm compresses. An otolaryngologist, who can examine your child's ears, nose, and throat with specialized tools to determine what's wrong, may be recommended to you by your primary care physician. They'll be able to identify any structural problems, like a deviated septum, that might make a child more prone to sinus problems.

## Allergies.

If your child's cough is accompanied by runny nose, itchy eyes, occurs at the same time every year, or occurs after each visit to Grandma and her two dogs, allergies may be to blame. They are merely the body's overreaction to an allergen, which is typically harmless to most people. Depending on the allergen, allergic rhinitis may be seasonal (possibly brought on by pollen from trees, weeds, grasses, and outdoor molds) or perennial (caused by year-round indoor allergens like dust mites, pets, and indoor molds).

**Symptoms:** Allergens cause the release of histamine and other biochemical compounds, which in turn cause inflammation and congestion, chronic postnasal drip, and a persistent, chronic cough in children.

**Treatment:** Nasal spray with saline solution or an over-the-counter antihistamine may help to reduce nasal secretions. A medical professional may advise corticosteroid or antihistamine nasal sprays if that doesn't relieve symptoms after a day or two. Avoid using over-the-counter decongestants and cough medications. While a chronic cough can be a sign of nasal allergies, experts say there is no evidence that these drugs are effective in treating coughs, and they occasionally exacerbate symptoms.

**The Best Allergy Drugs and Treatments for Children.**
Try to keep your child inside in the morning when pollen counts are at their highest if you suspect seasonal allergies are the culprit. There are several measures you can take to allergy-proof your home to help you fight a dust-mite allergy:.

• Purchase a pillow filled with polyester/fiber, not down feathers.

• Use covers that are dust-mite proof for the pillows and mattress.

• Launder bedding once per week.

• Regularly clean stuffed animals.

• Use a fan rather than a air conditioner.

• Use a dehumidifier, and make sure to change the filters often!

• Abstain from smoking.

The fumes from smoking remain on your clothing even if you smoke outside and will aggravate a cough. The same is true for vape pens or electronic cigarettes.

If none of these treatments relieves the cough, you should consult an allergist or immunologist who can perform a kid-friendly scratch test to identify the precise cause. Nasal allergies can cause chronic sinusitis, ear infections, sleep issues, asthma, and may hinder speech and language development if left untreated. Immunotherapy is a course of shots (for up to several years, depending on how well your child responds) that gradually improves the immune system's capacity to ward off allergy symptoms if your child is older than 5 and has not responded to conventional therapies.

**Asthma.**

Children who have asthma frequently experience chronic coughing. Asthma is a respiratory condition that affects the small airways in the lungs. An upper respiratory infection, allergens inhaled, irritants like secondhand smoke, cold and dry air, exercise, and even a temper tantrum can cause symptoms.

Wheezing, shortness of breath, chest pain, and coughing are possible symptoms for your child.

111

Typically, asthmatic kids can't get their coughs to stop.

But not all asthmatic children cough or gasp for air. Most people with asthma only have a chronic cough, which medical professionals usually refer to as cough-variant asthma. Due to the possibility that the results of standard diagnostic tests to measure lung capacity will be normal or because the child may be too young (under 6 years old) to properly perform the breathing test, this can go unnoticed for years.

Treatment: The medical professional will inquire about your child's symptoms, including any history of eczema or recurrent ear infections as a baby. Pulmonary function tests may be carried out by the medical professional to ensure that your child's lungs are healthy if they are old enough. When all of these symptoms are present, a health care provider may suspect that your child has asthma. Pay attention to what causes the cough, such as allergy season, whether they start to feel short of breath after just five minutes of playing soccer, and whether they awaken in the middle of the night with an uncontrollable cough.

## Toddler Cough: Reasons, Care, and When to Be Concerned.

Whether it is cough-variant or classic asthma, it typically responds to the same medications: bronchodilators and/or anti-inflammatory drugs. One is a "rescue" drug for when an attack (or fit of coughing) starts, and the other is a daily drug that "controls" the disease.

## Coughing up blood.

Pertussis, also known as whooping cough, is an extremely contagious bacterial respiratory illness.

**Symptoms:** Runny nose and sneezing are the first signs of whooping cough, which is then followed by brief fits of uncontrollable coughing that occasionally end with an audible whoop. Children who are struggling to breathe may vomit and turn blue. According to Dr. Berger, it's frequently called the "100-day cough.".

**Treatment:** Make an urgent phone call to a doctor because your child needs antibiotics. They can be given to additional family members later to stop the spread of the illness, but they are most effective when given within the first seven days of infection. Older children and adults with pertussis may only have a mild cough, but in infants who are too young to be immunized or who haven't received all doses of DTaP (a vaccine that also protects against tetanus and diphtheria), pertussis can have life-threatening consequences. Tdap is the whooping cough booster that pregnant women must receive between the 27th and 36th week of each pregnancy, as well as adults who frequently interact with young children.

# You Should Never Ignore These 12 Symptoms in Children.

Babies can't express heartburn, but GERD can cause them to gag, spit up, or act fussy while being fed. Older children may cough and wheeze, especially at night when they are lying down, or report chest or throat pain. A pediatric gastroenterologist may be consulted in order to diagnose GERD in children. GERD is typically diagnosed based on a history of symptoms and trial-and-error lifestyle changes.

**Treatment:** To lessen persistent coughing, keep infants upright for 30 minutes after feeding and raise the head of a child's mattress. Reduce the amount of foods, such as citrus fruits, tomatoes, chocolate, peppermint, and anything spicy, that older children typically consume to reduce the likelihood of GERD symptoms. Keep track of what your child consumes to determine if there is a connection. Reduce the amount of foods known to cause the condition and try not to feed older children right before bed.

**Tic or "Habit Cough.".**
It is particularly challenging to identify and treat a "habit cough.". Usually brought up after all other logical diagnoses have been ruled out. Perhaps your child's characteristic cough was brought on by a cold or the flu. The cough persists despite the fact that the cold has passed, with the

exception of while they sleep. Tics
can occasionally be brought on by
anxiety and develop into habits.
Children sometimes simply
develop the habit of coughing to
clear their throats. They continue
it if it garners attention.

**Treatment:** It might be sufficient
to reassure a child that they are no
longer ill. It might be necessary to
get a doctor to say this. However,
coughing itself can irritate the
throat and start a cycle of repeated
coughing. Offer a child who is
experiencing a coughing fit a sip of
water, a lollipop, or, for older
children, a cough drop to help
them stop coughing. In the event
that they don't cough,
compliments and reinforcement
are helpful. Pediatric

pulmonologists may instruct relaxation techniques to manage tics. If nothing helps, speak with a child therapist to determine if there is a deeper problem that needs to be addressed, such as a school phobia, shyness, or bullying.

## Who Can Treat a Child's Chronic Cough?

Your first port of call for the majority of coughs is a primary care physician. They will advise trying both over-the-counter and prescription drugs, or they will refer you to one of the following professionals:

**Allergists:** These medical professionals can perform skin tests to identify the substances your child is allergic to. An

allergist may suggest a
pulmonologist for a more
thorough examination of the lungs
if the results of other tests are still
inconclusive, such as a lung
function test or a chest X-ray that
measure the pattern of airflow into
and out of the lungs.

Otolaryngologist (ENT): After
taking a thorough medical history,
an expert in ears, noses, and
throats will check your child's
sinuses and nose. They might
require surgery to treat chronically
infected tonsils, adenoids, or
sinuses.

## Coughing.

When you cough, you suddenly
and incredibly quickly (up to 100
miles per hour) expel air from
your lungs through your epiglottis.
Coughing is the body's method of

removing unwelcome irritants from the airways thanks to the powerful air force it produces. A number of things must happen in order for a cough to happen. First, a large opening of the vocal cords allows more air to enter the lungs. The abdominal and rib muscles contract as the epiglottis closes off the windpipe (larynx), which raises the pressure behind it. The air is forcedfully expelled as a result of the increased pressure, and as it rushes past the vocal cords, it makes a rushing sound. It becomes possible to breathe comfortably once more as a result of the rushing air dislodging the irritant.

Certain coughs are dry. Others are successful.

Coughing up mucus is a sign of a productive cough.

Phlegm or sputum are additional names for mucus.

Both acute and persistent coughs are possible.

A cold, the flu, or a sinus infection are the most common causes of acute coughs, which typically start suddenly. After three weeks, they usually disappear.

3 to 8 weeks pass between acute cough episodes.

Chronic coughs persist for over eight weeks.

**Causes.**

These are typical causes of coughing.

• Sinus or nose-related allergies.

• Emphysema or chronic bronchitis; asthma; and COPD.

• The typical cold and the flu.

• Lung diseases like acute bronchitis or pneumonia.

• Postnasal drip and a sinus infection.

• Gastroesophageal reflux disease (GERD).

Some additional factors are:

• ACE inhibitors (drugs for the treatment of kidney disease, heart failure, and high blood pressure).

• Use of other drugs, such as marijuana, or exposure to secondhand smoke while smoking cigarettes.

The lung cancer.

• Conditions affecting the lungs, such as bronchiectasis or interstitial lung disease.

• Occasionally, no identifiable cause is discovered.

**Care at Home.**
Make sure you are taking the medications your doctor has prescribed if you have asthma or another chronic lung disease.

Following are some suggestions
for reducing coughing:.

Try cough drops or hard candy if
you have a dry, ticklish cough. As
they can cause choking, never give
these to children under the age of
three.

To add moisture to the air and
relieve a dry throat, use a
vaporizer or take a steamy shower.

Drink plenty of liquids: By
thinning the mucus in your throat,
liquids make it simpler to cough it
up.

Avoid smoking and being around
people who are smoking.

You can purchase the following
medications on your own:.

Mucus can be broken up by
guaifenesin. For dosage

information, refer to the package. Don't take more than what is advised. If you take this medication, be sure to stay hydrated.

Decongestants ease postnasal drip and dry up a runny nose. If you have high blood pressure, consult your physician before taking decongestants.

Before giving children aged 6 years or younger an over-the-counter cough medicine, even if it is labeled for children, talk to your child's doctor. These medications are probably ineffective for children and can have negative side effects.

If you experience hay fever or other seasonal allergies:

When there are many airborne allergens present (typically in the morning), stay inside.

Use an air conditioner and keep the windows closed.

DON'T use fans that pull air in from the outside.

After being outdoors, take a shower and switch into new clothing.

If you suffer from allergies all year long, use dust mite covers on your pillows and mattress, use an air purifier, and stay away from furry pets and other allergy-inducing substances.

# Chronic cough complications.

Coughing repeatedly can get annoying. Even if it only lasts a couple of days, having a cough is not fun, but for some people, it can last much longer. Even though coughs are frequently not serious and are frequently brought on by illnesses like the flu or a cold, some people can develop chronic coughs.

## The loss of bladder control.

If you cough frequently, you might notice that holding your bladder becomes more and more challenging. As you frequently need to force the cough out, you put pressure on your stomach when you cough. You won't be paying much attention to anything else because your body will be preoccupied with coughing up the toxins. Because of this, you may be having trouble controlling your urination, which occasionally results in you dribbling a little while you cough.

Even though we are aware that it is unpleasant, this is completely normal for someone who is coughing frequently. If your cough is bothering you and showing no signs of going away, you should consult an ENT physician.

**Sleeping problems.**
Sleep issues are another complication that you might encounter. Your body may be trying to clear whatever needs to come up through your cough, which can keep you awake throughout the night and obstruct your sleep. As a result of not

getting the uninterrupted sleep your body requires throughout the night, you might start to feel exhausted. It's worth talking to an ENT to see if there is anything that can be done if it is beginning to affect your daily life.

They might be able to help you manage the cough better so that you can get a good night's rest even if there isn't necessarily a way to get rid of it right away.

## Breathing difficulties or wheezing.

The constant coughing may also cause you to wheeze or feel out of breath. Your body has to expend a lot of energy when you cough, especially if you do it frequently because it strains your lungs more than they should. You should be able to feel the sensation where you are wheezing if you hear yourself wheezing, which typically comes from your chest. If this is occurring, you should schedule a consultation with an ear, nose, and throat specialist as soon as possible because it may be a sign of another issue.

When you cough frequently, you may also experience shortness of breath. When you cough, a lot of oxygen is used up, and you might feel as though you're having trouble breathing. Another clear indication that you should consult an ENT is that there might be a solution they can recommend to address this.

## Hoarseness.

If you are coughing constantly, this can irritate your vocal cords and cause mild laryngitis; have you noticed that your voice has changed somewhat? Your vocal cords will be inflamed because of this condition, which will alter the sound of your voice. To keep your throat comfortable and prevent any further problems from developing, make sure you are drinking plenty of fluids throughout the day.

## Nasal Vein Rupture.

Many people seem to forget that the throat, nose, and ears are all interconnected, and that symptoms can originate in any of these areas. If you are coughing frequently, the added pressure on your body could lead to vein ruptures in your nose. Keep an eye out for a nosebleed if this occurs. Before this occurs, you'll probably feel pressure around your eyes or even in your nose, which is a sign that you might soon be experiencing a nosebleed.

When treated at home, some coughs get better. To ascertain whether certain symptoms are a sign of a more serious problem, however, some must be evaluated quickly.

If you have a cough and are worried, think about going to urgent care.

The following types of coughs are frequently seen in emergency rooms:

**Headache caused by cough.**

- Persistent cough.
- Dry cough that lasts up to a week.
- Coughing up blood, mucus, or phlegm.
- A cough that does not respond to over-the-counter medications such as cough suppressants.

You should seek diagnosis if you have a cough that is accompanied by any of the following symptoms

Breathing problems such as wheezing, gasping, or shallow breathing.

- Chest pain.
- Malaise.

- Fever.

Body aches, chills, and vomiting are symptoms or signs of COVID-19.

What help can I get from my urgent care provider?

Discussing treatment options is one of the main reasons people visit urgent care centers.

According to Dr. Even, "We make suggestions that will help the patient get the best outcome and perhaps get rid of the cough quickly. Cough medicines and other treatments may also be part of the treatment for those who are not feeling well.

Another reason to visit an urgent care facility is to determine if the

cough is caused by a serious
medical condition. These include:

- Asthma.
-  Bronchitis.
- COVID-19.
- Croup.
- Pneumonia.
- Respiratory syncytial virus
  (RSV).
- Whooping cough.
- Use eucalyptus oil to avoid
  colds and coughs.

**Luca Coutinho.**
Are you worried about your child
catching a seasonal cold or cough
with the arrival of winter?
Eucalyptus, with its therapeutic
properties, can provide relief.
Read more.

Eucalyptus Oil Can Be Used to
Prevent Colds and Coughs

**Eucalyptus Essential Oil.**
A good source of wood, paper, and
essential oil is the fast-growing
eucalyptus tree.

Even though eucalyptus is native
to the Australian continent, it is
widely grown in tropical and
temperate regions of the world,
including the Americas, Europe,
Africa, the Mediterranean, the
Middle East, China, and the
Indian subcontinent. The
eucalyptus tree is called nilgiri in
India.

Eucalyptus essential oil has long
been used for its medicinal
properties. It is a powerful natural
antiseptic with anti-inflammatory,

antibacterial, antiviral, and antifungal properties that help treat a variety of conditions, including colds, coughs, wounds, boils, acne, insect bites, and skin infections.

**How is eucalyptus oil made?**
Eucalyptus oil is made by steam distillation after the leaves of the tree are dried, crushed, and the essential oil is extracted. The extracted oil is diluted and used as a topical application. Eucalyptus oil is the cure for colds and coughs.

We have all tried home remedies, over-the-counter medications, and prescription drugs in our battle against the common cold. But few people know that eucalyptus oil can be used to treat a variety of winter ailments, not just colds, coughs, and sore throats. Chest congestion, bronchial asthma, and sinusitis are just some of them. In general, eucalyptus is the best treatment for respiratory problems.

## Uses of eucalyptus oil include the following

Eucalyptus oil can be infused by placing a few drops in a small bowl of hot water to relieve chest congestion. Close your eyes, lower your head toward the bowl, and cover with a towel. Slowly inhale the steam containing eucalyptus. Place a few drops of oil on a hand towel lightly soaked in warm water and inhale the steam. To ease breathing, unclog sinuses, loosen mucus in the chest, and de-purge the area.

**WARNING** Adult supervision is required, even for older children.

Physical use is also possible: application of eucalyptus oil to the chest can further relieve coughs and congestion. In fact, along with other cough suppressants, some over-the-counter products known to relieve chest congestion contain about one point two percent eucalyptus oil.

## Commonly used terms include.

In aromatherapy, eucalyptus oil can be added to a diffuser to fill a space with the oil's natural aroma. Stress and fatigue are reduced.

Eucalyptus oil can be used as a mouthwash in addition to brushing your teeth twice a day to maintain oral health. Eucalyptus oil has antibacterial properties that help to eliminate oral bacteria, reduce plaque, and prevent gum disease.

Mix a very small amount of eucalyptus oil in a mouthwash and use it as a rinse. Even regular toothpaste can be made more effective by adding just a drop. In all cases, do not swallow mouthwash or paste. Spit it out after rinsing.

As an insect repellent. Cineole, the active ingredient in eucalyptus oil, is also the source of eucalyptus oil's strong scent. Natural insect repellent.

## Effectively repels insects and bugs.

As a result, it can be used to prevent insect-borne diseases such as dengue fever and malaria. Add a few drops of eucalyptus oil to water in a spray bottle. Use the spray to repel flies, mosquitoes, and other insects. Care should be taken not to use more than the advised amount of eucalyptus oil. It is very important to follow the directions and seek medical advice before using the oil, as there is always the possibility of overdose with the use of just a few drops.

# How to use honey for cough suppression.

Although honey does not completely eliminate coughing, there is some evidence that a single ingestion at bedtime can suppress coughing in infants. Honey soothes inflamed mucous membranes, coats the throat, calms coughs, and reduces associated symptoms.

In fact, according to some studies, honey appears to be as effective at suppressing nighttime coughs in children as dextromethorphan (found in cough syrups such as Robitussin for Children and Delsym Children's Cough Suppressant).

Honey has long been used as a traditional remedy for sore throats and coughs in both children and adults. It can be added to tea, warm lemon water, or taken by the teaspoon.

## HOW TO USE

Honey can be used alone or in combination with other cough medicines. It is a treatment without the risk of drug interactions, which is another advantage, in addition to being easy to obtain and affordable (in contrast to some over-the-counter medications used for the same purpose).

With the exception of those who are allergic to honey or have difficulty swallowing, almost all adults can use honey to relieve a cough. However, due to the risk of botulism, a rare form of poisoning brought on by a toxin that attacks the nervous system, honey should not be given to infants under 12 months.

## Honey may contain the soil bacterium botulinum.

The baby's digestive system is too immature to process these spores and as a result, the bacteria may multiply and produce toxins in the intestinal tract.

As a result, the bacteria may multiply and produce toxins in the intestinal tract. In adults, this can occur even though the majority of the digestive system can handle these spores. Immediate treatment is needed, as this can cause respiratory distress and muscle weakness.

## How to treat a cough with honey.

One to two teaspoons of honey may be taken as is, spread on toast, or with tea or lukewarm water. Even though honey can be consumed as needed, it is still a good source of calories and sugar. The American Heart Association recommends limiting sugar intake to about 30 grams per day, so try to keep your daily honey intake to no more than 6 teaspoons.

# Three ways to use ginger to prevent and treat coughs and colds.

Ginger is rich in both anti-inflammatory and immune-boosting properties.

Because ginger is a hot, spicy herb, it also provides the heat that the body needs at this time of year to relieve the pain associated with a sore throat.

Anti-inflammatories also help to soothe a sore throat.

In addition, they prevent those infections by boosting the immune system. Thus, if you have a sore throat, cough, or cold-like symptoms, ginger can be your first line of defense.

## Ginger and Honey-Based Drinks

A sore throat is the first warning sign that the flu or other infection has taken hold in the body. Grate ginger and add it to boiling water.

When boiling, add honey and finish with a squeeze of half a lemon.

It works well for coughs and sore throats.

For sore throats, ginger reduces inflammation caused by irritation, while honey helps soothe the throat while reducing the frequency of dry coughs. Ginger and Lemon.

Mixing ginger and lemon juice in warm water can prevent and expel phlegm from the body. In addition, ginger has antioxidant properties and helps the body get rid of toxins, thus helping the body get rid of infections and flu. Add lemon juice to boiled ginger water.

In addition to helping to expel mucus and relieve pain, the vitamin C in the lemon also acts as an active ingredient.

**Ginger and Tulsi.**
For a very long time this was one of the most popular remedies in Indian homes.

To make the tea, simply grate the ginger and add four to five Tulsi leaves to the water. After boiling for a minute or so, add the rest of the ingredients. If you have a fever, drinking this ginger and tulsi infusion will reduce the fever.

It also helps relieve headaches and coughs.

**Chamomile tea is used for cough relief.**
Chamomile tea, known for its healing properties, has been used for insomnia, back pain, and anxiety. However, its most typical use is as a muscle relaxant. Consult a physician before using herbal remedies to treat symptoms to avoid allergic reactions. Chamomile tea reduces inflammation and relieves menstrual cramps and other body aches. Pregnant women should not drink chamomile tea.

**Citrus.**

If a cough is caused by a virus or bacteria, vitamin C can prevent infection by strengthening the immune system. Citrus fruits such as lemons and oranges are not only rich in vitamin C, but are also thought to help clear mucus from the throat. Mix a teaspoon of vitamin C with your meals to get a healthy dose. Per cup of hot chamomile tea or lemon or orange juice.

**Ginger.**

According to the University of Maryland Medical Center, ginger root herb may reduce inflammation, such as bronchial and throat irritation, and relieve sore throats caused by colds and flu. Steep and drink 2 tablespoons of something to soothe a cough. Add 1 teaspoon of freshly grated ginger root to 2 cups of hot chamomile tea. Consult a physician before using this herbal remedy, as ginger has been found to have blood thinning properties and may interact with medications such as aspirin.

**Other Health Benefits**
Chamomile tea has been demonstrated to have antibacterial, anti-inflammatory, sedative, and antispasmodic properties, in addition to its ability to reduce cough symptoms. According to the American Chemical Society, hippurate, a component of chamomile tea, enhances the body's defense

mechanisms. Despite the fact that chamomile is often consumed as a beverage, several topical remedies containing ingredients from the chamomile flower may also be effective for skin inflammation. Another benefit of drinking chamomile tea is that it reduces painful muscle contractions, especially in the uterus and intestines. For this reason, chamomile tea is effective in treating diarrhea, irritable bowel syndrome, indigestion, and menstrual cramps.